Fine-ly Fabulous!

A Survival Guide for the Fine-Haired Girl

Caren Cantrell
Melissa Glass

First Printing, 2011
Second Printing, 2015

102nd Place, LLC

Printed in the United States of America

TABLE OF CONTENTS

LET'S GET FABULOUS!

Stringy, lifeless, limp, flat, and greasy – are these the words you use to describe your hair? Would you rather be using words like luscious, plump, full, and healthy? Well now you can. Melissa and Caren have put their combined fabulous, fine-haired heads together to give you all the secrets you need!

The Law of Abundance

If any of you have been paying attention to the self-help gurus and motivational speakers lately, you already know about the Law of Abundance. Basically it says that there is more than enough health, wealth, happiness, prosperity and (fill in the blank) in the universe than could ever be consumed by everyone on the planet. All you have to do is think positive thoughts about what it is you desire and it will come to you. For example, if you stop weighing yourself daily and keep thinking of yourself as already being at your ideal weight, then the law of abundance says that your body will naturally take you to that weight. So theoretically you could argue that all you really need to do to get that great head of hair that you've always wanted is to think positively about it and think about it as if you already have it. If you are sincere in your efforts then one day you should wake up with thick, fabulous hair.

And why not – go for it! But while you're waiting with your positive thoughts and imagery we think you should also practice another little law that many of us grew up with - that God or the Universe or Who/Whatever helps those that help themselves. And that's where this book comes in.

Defining Fine

Let's start by defining what fine is and what it's not. Many people assume that fine is synonymous with thin. But that's not the case. Fine refers to the diameter of a single strand of hair. The smaller the diameter of the strands, the finer the hair will be. You can have fine hair even though you have full hair. Fine and full hair means that you have small diameter strands but you have a lot of them per square inch on your head. Fine and thin on the other hand means not only is the strand small in diameter but you don't have very many strands per square inch either. A double whammy!

The Masters of Illusion

We've all heard of the great masters of illusion but probably the greatest of our time is David Copperfield. He has been thrilling audiences for years with his magic. Most notably back in 1986 when he made the Statue of Liberty disappear before our very eyes! He was able to "trick" us all by using a series of optical illusions. An optical illusion is defined as a visually perceived image that differs from objective reality. And magic is simply creating illusions of seemingly impossible feats, using purely natural means. The same can be said of truly great fine-hair stylists. They are our own private masters of illusion.

Getting the right cut, adding the right color in the right amount in the right place, and using the right tools and products are all the ways that a stylist can "trick" the eye and create the illusion of full, lustrous, fabulous hair. It's all about attracting the eye to what you want it to see and fooling the brain that what the eye is seeing is in fact what exists. For this reason finding an experienced illusionist (hair stylist) is so important that we've devoted an entire chapter to it! Then in chapters 4, 5 and 6 we'll let you in on the "tricks" of the trade specifically designed with the fine-haired girl in mind.

And just like David Copperfield or Houdini or any of the other great illusionists, sometimes tricking the eye requires the use of props. In our case, think wigs, extensions, head bands, or an appropriately placed barrette. You'll find a chapter on these as well.

An illusionist is only as good as the materials he/she has to work with. Keeping the hair you have, whether fine and full or fine and thin, healthy and in great shape can take your illusion from the vaudeville stage to Madison Square Garden. So in the last chapter we talk about diet and nutrition. We also focus on some of the more successful hair restoration techniques in case that ever becomes an issue.

So let's get started, shall we? It's time for you to become Fine-ly Fabulous!

FALLING IN LOVE WITH FINE

The Zen of Hair

No one told Melissa in cosmetology school that cutting and styling hair would only be about 5% of the job. Or that the other 95% would require a degree in psychology with a minor in social work! They never warned her that many of her clients would likely have a vision of what they would look like under her artistry that would not be remotely close to what she would be able to produce. Of course deep down she knew – after all hadn't she spent the majority of her own life under that same delusion?

We women obsess about our hair. We agonize over how to style it, to go short or long, natural or highlights, curly or straight and on and on. We worry that whatever we decide our mothers, husbands, boyfriends and even our bosses won't approve. We'd like to think that hairstyles are just fun and fashionable but experts say they send a message about our identity to others. In fact, the topic of hair and self-image is so important, it is the total focus of the book "Rapunzel's Daughters: What Women's Hair Tells Us About Women's Lives" by Rose Weitz.

Hair is one of the first things that people notice about us. As Ms. Weitz recounts it has been used throughout time to convey messages about our age, gender, politics, social-class, and more. When we cut our hair short, dye it or let it go gray, we decide what image we want to project to the world. Others judge us and respond to us partly because of our hair and it's these responses that help shape our identities and ultimately our feelings of worth. In 2001, Hillary Rodham Clinton, whose hairdos are constantly analyzed, told the Yale graduating class:

"Your hair will send significant messages to those around you: what hopes and dreams you have for the world, but more, what hopes and

dreams you have for your hair. Pay attention to your hair, because everyone else will."

Hair can play a large part in a woman's confidence and in their success in relationships and in the workplace, either boosting or tearing down her self esteem. We rely heavily on our appearance to make a positive impression on others. According to information developed by the Federal Reserve Bank of St. Louis, workers with below average looks tend to earn an average of 9% less per hour than above average looking workers. The last thing we want to do is look in the mirror and see that our childhood cowlick has decided to make a mid-life reappearance or that we're only one shade away from matching colors with a popular restaurant's star clown! When we feel that our hair isn't up to par we tend to feel insecure in our abilities and it shapes our entire day. If we feel like our hair looks good it's a psychological boost.

The end line is the better our hair looks, the better we feel. The better we feel, the more confident we are. The more confident we are, the more successful we'll be. Such is the power that our hair holds over us. Understanding this power and using it to finally end our struggles for perfection is the key to creating inner happiness. Accepting and celebrating our own unique "head-topping" gives us ultimate power. Controlling our hair means controlling our lives.

Making Peace and Letting Go

Unfortunately, most women are disappointed in their own hair. A 2003 Pantene survey found that 84% of women wish they could improve their hair's appearance. And for those of us with thin or fine hair the percentage is even higher. Consequently, we are always searching for the ONE miracle stylist, product, or tool that will make our hair look and feel like those sirens on the tiny screen with long, luxurious, silky locks. And we'll pay almost anything to find it!

We once read of a stylist who actually kept a "magic wand" at his station. When clients would come in with requests for cuts or color to look like some super model or movie star he would literally take the wand, tap them on the head and say, "Not unless this wand will produce a miracle." The point is that much of what we see on television or in magazines isn't real. Those actresses and models, even the ones we know, have all been air-brushed or digitally mastered to look perfect. We can't BE these people; heck they can't even be these people! It's all an illusion.

But that doesn't mean we can't put our best "fine hair" forward each and every day. We just have to let go of that image of thick, infinitely manageable, totally versatile hair that Madison Ave. wants us to lust after and learn how to love our own unique locks. We need to let go of the fear that has kept us wearing our hair the same way we did in high school. 80% of us do you know! There are miracles to be had. They start with being realistic about what naturally works and what doesn't. They start with finding the right stylist who understands how to work with thin/fine hair and who isn't afraid to tell you when what you are asking he or she to do is not going to produce the results you want. And they start with you truly believing that your hair can and will look fabulous!

MY HAIR LADY (OR MAN)

Few things are more important to a woman than finding a stylist that they like and trust. Over the years your stylist tends to become one of your BFFs (best friends forever)! Once you find someone who understands you and your hair you'll follow that person to the ends of the earth. We know one client who followed her stylist from one salon to another for over 20 years until finally the client moved out of town. Even then she tried for a while to time her haircuts and colors around visits back home. Only when that stopped being an option did she finally turn her sights toward finding a new stylist.

Beginning the Search

So you're in a new town and you hardly know anyone, how do you start finding a new stylist? Or you're tired of the way you've been wearing your hair but your current stylist wants you to like them more than they want to risk you not liking a new cut or color. The very thought of finding someone new can cause sweaty palms and a rapid heart beat. Well, relax! Here are a few easy tips to get you started.

1. Talk to people you meet who have healthy shiny hair or a hair cut or style that you particularly like. These can be people at work, at the gym, at your church or just standing in the grocery line. Ask them who they use and what salon they are at. Don't worry about being too nosey. Women are flattered when someone wants to know who does their hair and are more than willing to assist. Ask for the phone number if they have it or better yet their stylist's business card. And don't forget to ask them for their name as well! Many stylists give special bonuses to clients who refer other clients.

2. Do some research on the web. You can find out a lot about the stylist and the salon she/he is associated with by doing a simple Google search. Be sure when putting in the

stylist's name that you include the city or the state in which they work to narrow your search. Look to see if the salon fits your needs. Is it located near work or home? Are the hours convenient? Do they have other services that you would use? You can often tell if a particular stylist is going to be out of your price range by looking at the salon's website. Does the stylist have any customer reviews and if so, are they positive.

3. Book a consultation! Never, **NEVER**, just go in and have someone start working on your hair! This is a recipe for disaster and at today's prices can be a very expensive mistake. If the stylist is any good, a consultation is as much to her/his benefit as it is to yours. And as a test run, ask for a shampoo and blow out to really get an idea of their skill working with fine or thin hair.

The Art of Consultation

Asking a stylist for a consultation as a potential new client is standard practice. A good consultation sets the tone for your entire relationship, and you know how important that is. Remember BFF? If a stylist you select doesn't do consultations then don't waste your time or money. It's obvious she/he isn't interested in listening to your concerns or challenges up front which means she/he most likely won't listen when you're in the chair either. Find a different stylist!

Most salons and stylists don't charge for a consultation. Therefore, you should strive to keep the consult between 10 to 15 minutes since you are asking them for time that they could be spending on a paying client. That simply means you need to be prepared when you go to the consultation to ask pertinent questions that will help you make an informed decision about becoming a client. Here are some of the questions you should ask:

1. Ask about their experience.

How long have they been doing hair? If they are fresh out of cosmetology school then you may not want to take the risk. However, if the price is right and you like everything else giving a new person some experience could be a win-win.

How long have they been working at this salon? If it's less than a year follow up by asking where they worked previously and why they left. Bouncing from salon to salon without a valid reason may be a sign that they don't do good work or that they aren't reliable.

When was the last education class or training conference they attended, and what did they learn? A good stylist should always be educating themselves about the latest technologies and trends in the hair industry by attending classes to fine-tune their craft. If the stylist isn't keeping up with education it could mean that your hair style will be stuck in the 70's, 80's or 90's as well!

2. Ask about their work.

Do they specialize in fine or thin hair?

Do they specialize in curly or straight, short or long?

What types of products do they use? Are there any that may be a problem for you?

If you are interested in having the stylist do color as well as cut, ask how they will help you determine the right color for you. If you are looking to add "warmth" to your hair – ask the stylist to show you in a color book what warmth means to them. It will help you to ensure that you are communicating accurately and both have the same definitions.

Do they have a "look" book that you can review to see what they have done for other clients?

If you are still unsure, is the stylist comfortable referring you to their clients who have similar hair challenges?

Other Consultation Tips

Since the consultation is for the benefit of both you and the stylist, do come with a scrapbook and/or pictures of cuts/color that you like and dislike. Include pictures of yourself at times when you really did and did not like your hair cut and/or color. There can be a lot of confusion when interpreting words used to describe hair styles so having a picture helps the stylist know if she/he can do what you need. Be realistic about what your hair will or will not do. Remember those magazine models are deceiving with hair extensions, lighting and air brushing!

Look around the salon during the consult. Is it too busy or not busy enough? How are the stylists dressed? How do they do their hair? If you are more conservative and you see stylists and clients who have "alternative" hairstyles then this salon is probably not a good fit. Is the salon clean with a relaxed, comfortable atmosphere? Was the receptionist friendly and responsive? Do the stylists appear to be happy?

Have the stylist recap the consultation. This will be your opportunity to clear up any misunderstandings. It is also an opportunity for the stylist to tell you what kind of hair care plan she/he would like to put in place for you. **Do Not** ask the stylist about fees for services. This question should be asked of the receptionist at the end of the consult. Less expensive could mean less experience, but understand that pricing may also differ based on the local market. You want a good value.

And Then There Was One

So you've done your due diligence and been through the consultation and you've narrowed it down to **THE ONE**. The next step is of course to take the plunge and schedule an appointment. Here we go again, sweaty palms and rapid heart beats. Just keep in mind that even with a perfect fit it may take one or two appointments for your new stylist to get to know exactly how that little cowlick in your bangs works, and which shade of honey yellow makes your blue eyes pop! Give her a chance. After all, you've just met your new BFF!

A CUT ABOVE

Face the Music

Nothing says "wow" quite like a great hairstyle. But even a well executed and well cut hairstyle can spell disaster if it's performed on the wrong face shape. The reason is that hairstyles are all about geometry and balance. Your hairstyle needs to frame your face so that a perfect balance between brow, cheekbones and jawline occurs. It needs to minimize your not so great features and promote and compliment the positive ones. There is a general rule that your hairstyle should be designed and balanced to achieve an oval face shape. The oval is considered the perfect shape because it is the most pleasing to the human eye. Look at the models and film stars who are considered real beauties; most likely they have oval face shapes.

A great hairstylist, like the one you just picked in Chapter 3, should instinctively know what type hairstyle will or won't suit you. However, you should also understand face shape and hairstyle because it will allow you to communicate better with your stylist. You'll have confidence that when she says a particular cut or style won't work based on the shape of your face that she's really got your best interest at heart and not avoiding a complicated cut.

There are seven basic types of face shapes:

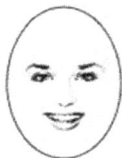

Oval – ideal shape because it is longer than it is wide and appears balanced

Styles that work:
>   Lucky, lucky you! Women with an oval shaped face can wear any length of hair (short, long, layered or bobbed) and any style
>   The only thing you need to consider is what part of your face you want to accentuate

<u>Styles to steer clear of:</u>
Avoid styles that make your hair fall into your face or eyes or in general cover up your naturally perfect shape

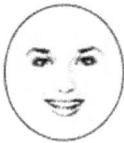

Round – face is as wide as it is long with, soft round edges

<u>Styles that work:</u>
Styles that are very short or that fall below the chin work well
Any style that minimizes volume around the face; layering should be done at the top of the head in order to add length to the face
Hair that is swept back can also make a round face look narrower as can using a middle part
Side swept bangs are also a good look

<u>Styles to steer clear of:</u>
Anything that adds volume through the sides such as curly short hair, cropped or chin-length bob cuts
Side parts and heavy straight across bangs create a wider, shorter shape and should be

avoided if your hairstyle does not include a lot of height on top

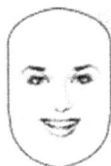

Square – brow bone, cheekbone and jawline are approximately the same width; face is as wide as it is long but with more of an angular appearance than a round face. Aim is to soften your strong jawline.

Styles that work:
Short to medium hair looks best
For longer hair, go for layers that start at the jaw and work their way down with wispy ends that fall forward onto your face
Curly or wavy styles are also good choices as they give a more rounded look

Styles to steer clear of:
Chin length bobs
Middle parts
Straight heavy bangs

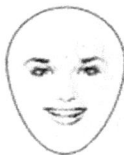

Heart – has a narrow jaw and is wider at the forehead and/or cheekbones. Goal should be to add some length to the shape and create width around the chin

Styles that work:

Bobs are a great way to balance a heart shaped face

If you use bangs make sure they are side swept to draw attention to your eyes and away from your chin

Shoulder length cuts with wispy ends that kick out

Styles to steer clear of:

Anything with choppy layers; layers must be long to look balanced

Super short hair or hair that is slicked back from the face

Volume or height on top only works with shoulder length or longer hair

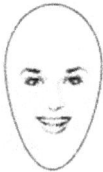

Diamond – defined by short, angular lines. The cheekbones are noticeably wider than the brow bones. Goal should be to shorten the overall length of the face and balance the narrow chin by narrowing the cheekbones.

Styles that work:

Same as for a heart shaped face

Also try styles that tuck in behind the ears to show off the cheekbones
Side parts
Straight across bangs work well to shorten the face

Styles to steer clear of:
Short hairstyles that have a lot of height on top; particularly if they are without bangs
Middle parts because they add length
Short styles that leave no hair on the neck area or around the chin

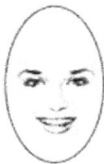

Oblong – face is longer than it is wide so obviously the goal is to add width to minimize the vertical length.

Styles that work:
Short or medium length
Longer top layers without height
Brow skimming straight across bangs
Chin length or shoulder length with ends that turn under or kick out with thick hair on the sides of the face
Side parts

Layered cuts with wavy and curly textures in medium to long lengths

Styles to steer clear of:
Middle parts as these add length
Styles without bangs
Styles that don't add body or width through the sides
Volume and height at the top or the crown of the head

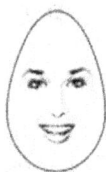

Triangular – face becomes progressively wider from the brow bone to the jawline. The objective here is to narrow the chin and widen the forehead.

Styles that work:
Layers on top or the upper part of the face
Styles that involve tucking the hair behind the ears
Styles that create fullness at the temples
Shorter works best

Styles to steer clear of:
Longer lengths, particularly those that hit just below the jawline

Straight blunt bobs
Any style that draws attention to
your chin area

It's Just a Number Right?

Your age that is. Aren't we only as old as
we feel? Shouldn't our hair reflect our
youthful outlook no matter our age?

Unfortunately when it comes to age, your
hair refuses to be fooled. In addition to its
chronological age (the actual time it's spent
on your head), your hair also has a
"hormonal" age. As if adolescence and
puberty weren't enough, hormonal aging
occurs as a result of the physical changes
that we lucky women experience as we
grow older. These hormonal impacts result
in reduced melanin production which is
our hair's natural protection and defense
mechanism. It also results in slowed scalp
activity which means our hair doesn't
replace as quickly as before. I know – it's
just another nail in the coffin of the girl
with fine/thin hair.

There are six signs of age damaged hair:
graying, dullness, increased dryness,
changes in texture, thinning, and breakage.

If you've ever wondered why most women as they age tend to keep cutting their hair shorter and shorter, hormonal aging is a key factor. Shorter hair simply looks better and healthier than long hair when you're dealing with one or more age damage issues.

But that's not the only reason women cut their hair as they age. Let's face it our rear ends aren't the only things subject to the pull of gravity! Our faces react as well. As we age, unless we do a little nip/tuck, we are naturally going to see some sagging in the chin area and in general around the entire jawline. This causes the face to appear longer and as we learned earlier in this chapter the way to balance a longer face is to have shorter hair.

Compound the sagging with having fine hair that is also starting to thin and shorter just makes sense. Fortunately there have been so many advances in cuts, styling techniques and products that short no longer means boring. With the right cut and the right color we can still look as young as we feel!

I'm not saying that you absolutely have to give up your long hair if that's what you really want. Many women can and do pull it off every day. Whether or not you are one of those women will depend mainly on your hair's texture. If your hair is fine but you have a lot of it, then by all means let it all hang down!

Hair and Now

The type of hairstyle or cut that is right for you depends as much on your lifestyle as it does on the shape of your face. You can have the most perfect look in the world but if you don't have the time to wash, blow dry, or curl each day so that it looks exactly like it did when you left the salon then most of the time you may end up looking less than your best.

Everyone's lifestyle differs in a variety of ways and it's extremely important for you to talk about yours with your stylist before the scissors come out. Are you in a professional occupation by day but play in a grungy rock band at night? Are you a mother with small children with hardly any time to take a shower let alone work with your hair? Do you enjoy an athletic lifestyle but love to "glam it up" when you go out?

Talking about all of these things will help you and your stylist determine the right cut and style.

For example if you spend a lot of time participating in sporting events or you regularly work in a greasy restaurant and find yourself washing your hair on a daily basis then a style that is both short and convenient to wash and dry would be good for you. If you have absolutely no time to mess with your hair then you might want to try a wave or curly perm so that you can just scrunch and air dry.

It seems that for those of us with thin or fine hair many of the real challenges come when we decide to workout, hit the beach or go to the pool. Or really any activity that causes our hair to get wet without the benefit of products and blow dryers. Sure our hair looks great as we settle into our sand chairs or lounges and then as the day begins to heat up – the big dilemma strikes! Are we going to stay put sweating through the day or take the plunge and cool off knowing full well that our hair when it dries is going to look like something the cat drug in? Drowned rat anyone? Here are some tips to consider.

If your hair is medium to long:

1. Try braiding – make it interesting by doing a tiny braid on each side of your head starting at the crown and then melding those two braids into one at the back of your head.

2. Pull it back into a ponytail but be extremely careful of the band that you use. Scrunchies are great but not always in style. Elastic bands cause breakage even with thick hair so try to avoid these. If you must use an elastic band get ones with the thickest cloth around them for protection.

3. If you must pull back your hair, do so at the nape of your neck rather than at the top of your head. This will result in less tension on the hair and therefore, less breakage.

4. Also try twisting your hair before putting it in to a band and using a bobby pin between your hair and the band to help lessen the likelihood of breakage.

If your hair is short:

1. Consider getting a body perm and take some hair gel along with you. Then towel

dry, put in some gel and then sit and scrunch your hair up as it dries.

2. Bring a product with you like sea salt texturizer – spray it in when your hair is semi-dry and use your fingers as a back comb.

3. To add some volume – after your hair is dry or even as it is drying, use your hand to make a claw and use a circular motion at your scalp to lift the hair. Then gently smooth it over with the palm of your hand filling in the holes. This approach also works great for fixing cowlicks at any time of the day.

Of course it's always appropriate to use the old "hat trick" to manage the wet hair blues. A trendy hat is always in style and there are so many choices these days that it's pretty easy to find one that flatters your face. Head bands have also become very popular and can be used to enhance our wet dog look. Just be sure not to wear your headband in the same spot every day because they too can cause breakage.

There is another danger for fine, thin hair that comes along with most outdoor activities like biking, gardening, swimming, hiking, etc. It's sun damage. Sun exposure can make your hair look brassy or faded, particularly if you color it. So make sure your stylist knows if you spend a lot of time outdoors. She can use special products that extend your color's life and keep you from having to return too soon. The end line is to make sure your hairstyle suits your personality and your lifestyle.

GOODBYE LIMP – HELLO LUSCIOUS!

So now we have the right stylist and the right hair cut to match our face and lifestyle. All we need now is to go from flat to fabulous! Creating volume isn't as hard as you might think. With the right cut and color your stylist can easily make your hair appear 2 to 3 times fuller.

Start out with a volume enhanced haircut. This normally will entail layering of some sort. Again, make sure your stylist knows how to cut fine hair. An inexperienced stylist might leave scissor marks in your finished style. Beware of some razor cutting techniques on fine/thin hair. They can cause split ends and make hair too fly away. Again, experience reigns supreme so ask your stylist how often she cuts fine hair with a razor before agreeing to this technique. Baby bangs, those that fall only to the middle of the forehead, work well with fine hair but not if you have a receding hairline. A side swept bang gives the illusion of thickness and frames the face nicely.

I'm Home – Now What?

Everyone looks great when they step out of the salon. And you may even look great the next day if you sleep just so and you don't have to shampoo. But sooner or later we all have to face the dreaded day of reckoning when we try to reproduce the magic that our stylist so effortlessly performed. Don't sweat it! First of all, realize that not even your stylist can create the exact same effect as HER stylist when she gets home! Granted she might get close but let's face it, when you can't see the back of your head and you have your arms bent at unusual angles to get the brush and blow dryer in the right place at the right time – it can be a crap shoot! Most of us aren't ambidextrous so our only solution to get better is to practice, practice, practice. Oh, and using a few of these tips to take yourself from limp to LUSCIOUS!

1. Use a volumizing shampoo in the shower. There are quite a few products on the market that offer documented proof of ingredients that work to plump the hair shaft. Your stylist should be able to recommend a few including those sold in drug or grocery stores.

2. Skip using rinse out conditioners unless your hair is damaged, curly, or wavy. Most rinse out conditioners are too heavy for fine hair and will weigh it down. If you must use a rinse out conditioner try to find one that says it is "weightless" or specifically developed for fine hair. When using, only apply the conditioner from the middle of the shaft to the ends of the hair where the damage, curl or wave is most likely to be. Avoid using the conditioner at the root to minimize any weigh down effect.

3. Finish your hair off with a cool/cold rinse to close the cuticle shaft and add shine.

4. Towel dry hair. Use a spray leave in detangling conditioner sparingly. Using too much will cause hair to flatten just like a leave in conditioner would. Comb out

using a wide tooth comb to avoid pulling and breaking hair.

5. Use volume enhancing products at the roots to give maximum lift and separation. A root boost, either a mouse or spray will lift the roots and give volume. Use a spray gel or a light styling spray on the mid-shaft to the ends. Again, ask your stylist for recommendations. You may also want to air dry just a little to naturally build in a fuller look. Take this "air time" to get dressed or do your make-up.

6. Blow dry your hair using your fingers. Lift the hair up from the scalp while you dry to create volume. Some stylists believe you achieve extra fullness if you flip your hair over and dry upside-down. Others seem to think that this method creates flat spots on the head. You'll need to experiment to see what works best with your hair. In either case you should be "messy" drying, continuously moving the blow dryer while you lift your hair. At this point you are not trying to style the hair, just give it some lift.

7. When hair is damp (75-80% dry), turn your blow dryer on the low setting. Be careful not to "over-blow" the style. Take

the top section of your hair and pin it out of the way (where the head starts to roll). Section again at the temples and pin out of the way. It your hair is long, section again at the ear, and maybe one more section about 3 to 4 inches from the bottom hairline. It will be easier and faster to dry your hair by sectioning it out of your way. If your hair is short, only section at the top and the temples.

8. Use a round brush to add lift. The goal is to create volume. You may need to use 2 different sizes to get the best look. A small and medium sized brush works well. Get brushes that allow you to curl the hair around the brush not more than 1 ½ or 2 times. Anything more may result in tangling. Do your bangs first because if they don't get dried properly they will look funky and can be difficult to correct. For the rest of your hair, work your way from the bottom to the top.

You want to work in sections that are slightly smaller in width than the brush itself. If you are having trouble working with the brush, section, and blow dryer all at once, simply turn the blow dryer off and set it down. Section the hair you want to blow dry and anchor it in the brush. Then pick the blow dryer up, turn it on and work with that section. Continue this until your hair is dry. If this is new to you, don't get discouraged, just remember practice, practice, practice. You'll get the hang of it in no time. If your blow dryer has a cool button, use it to "set" the curl. Just think of hair like plastic. You heat it up to mold and shape it then cool it down to set it.

9. Here is a little trick to avoid a flat spot on the top of your head. Take the top section and divide it in two with one section that is on the very top near your part. Take this section and "over direct" your brush in the opposite direction. For example, if you are working a section on the right side of your head, instead of pulling the brush up from your scalp and then down the right side, pull the brush over to the left side of your head and dry then bring it back down over the right. When you roll it back it will be what is called "on base." This will prevent a flat spot near your part on the top your head.

10. Now that it's all dry, what do you do? Have you ever noticed that your hair may work better for you on the 2nd day? That's because some of the natural oils and products that your body produces give it

texture. When your hair is too clean it has a tendency to not hold a style so we need to dirty it up a little. Use a "texturizing spray" that contains sea salt to give it that day 2 feel. Messy spray the product in dry hair and hit it with the blow dryer. Afterwards, smooth into place with a metal pick. Your hair will look like you've spent the day at the beach.

Such a Tease

To backcomb, or not to backcomb, this is the question. Backcombing, or teasing for the more mature crowd, is a great way to create even more lift and volume and to "fill in" the holes. However, if not done properly you can cause breakage and damage.

Take a 1 inch section and hold it tight between the palm of your thumb and your fingers. Take a fine toothed comb and start 2 to 3 inches from scalp and pull comb down. Do this 3 to 4 times to create a "base." Repeat this procedure in 3 to 5 different spots. Then use a smoothing pick (metal works best as plastic is too thick) to lightly smooth over the top layer. You don't want the "base" to show, so look for holes and smooth with pick. If your hair is already damaged but you still need lift instead of backcombing, try using a light hairspray at the root and pinning it with a small metal clip until it dries.

So there you have it! Just because your hair is fine doesn't mean you have to live with limp. Utilizing these techniques will help you look and feel like one of those girls with thick "TV ad" hair. Remember to experiment and play around with your hair to see what works best for you. When you don't like the results simply rinse and repeat. And have some FUN!!!!

ANY COLOR WON'T DO

Remember back in grade school during art class how you were taught that colors could be used to make images stand out? How the right combination of light and dark colors would instantly give your picture that 3-dimensional look? How shading in the right places would add depth? Well it doesn't work for just art on a canvas. The right combination of colors can also give the illusion of depth (think volume) to your hair! When applied properly and artistically by a professional hair stylist you will get the appearance of fuller, thicker hair.

Thinking color may be your ticket to great hair? Follow this first rule: Never, Never, Never color fine/thin hair yourself at home. Coloring fine hair is tricky. It is more susceptible to over-processing, chemical damage and breakage. Not to mention that the age of the color you are using will have an impact on results. There is no easy way to tell how long that box of light auburn has been sitting on the shelf. If it's been there too long you may end up with something closer to Day-Glo orange!

A great color stylist knows how chemicals will interact and how to formulate color correctly to expand the diameter of the hair. They know how and where to place color to give the effect of fuller hair without causing damage.

Trip the Lights

Highlights and lowlights that is. Highlighting hair is a process that is done by coloring or bleaching strands of hair to lighten the hair to different tones. Lowlights are the opposite. Lowlights consist of adding a darker color for contrast creating depth and dimension. Adding highlights and lowlights gives hair more texture which is exactly what fine hair is lacking.

When all is said and done, you should be left with three different levels and shades of color in your hair – highlights, natural color, and lowlights. Lowlights are typically a shade or two darker than your natural color. But be careful, if they are too dark the color will look unnatural. Lowlights work well if your hair is starting to get too blonde and is losing depth. Lowlights also do not show re-growth as much since they typically blend with your natural color. Highlights are usually performed first and placed in foil packets to keep them away from other hair. Lowlights can either be "painted" in second or also put into foil packets.

Highlights and lowlights can be added in basically two ways. The first is to use foils. In this method, small sections of individual strands are placed on a foil and then the color is added with a special brush from the root to the end. The foil is then folded over the hair. Foils can only be done in a profes-sional salon setting. They add ribbons of color to the hair; give you the most control and generally the best results.

The second method is to use free hand hair painting called bialiage. Hair painting can be done with just a few strands or it can be done "chunky" which means that huge sections of strands are painted. If you've ever seen a young man or woman with big, trendy sweeps of purple or green in their hair, chances are they were done in "chunky" style.

Bialiage is great for women who may be a little skeptical about highlighting their hair and just want to try it out on a few areas. It is also good for women with very short hair as it will give you the most natural finish. Anyone who wants to exactly control where the color goes in their hair can use hair painting. As can someone who lets their color "grow out" and needs to get a more blended look. With bialiage you can get up to five different shades for a more natural look. This is perfect for the woman who has a wonderful natural color but just wants to add some subtle lighter shades.

One Color Wonder

Not everyone needs to use highlights and lowlights to add depth and the illusion of fullness to their hair. The same effect can be created with an all over color. In this case, you'll need to choose a color that is deep and rich. So if you only look fantastic as a platinum blonde then over all color may not be the right choice for you. However, if you have a great natural darker shade and you're just trying to cover up the annoying gray then this approach is perfect!

There are three different routes to go if you decide to do an all over color - permanent, semi-permanent, or demi-permanent. Permanent color is just that – permanent. It typically does not wash out, it has to grow out. Permanent color is most often used to cover gray.

If you are looking to stay at your natural level but want to change tone then you can use a semi-permanent. Semi-permanents gradually wash out after 6 weeks or so.

A demi-permanent is similar but has more staying power than a semi and won't wash out as fast. Regardless of type, an all over color will require a root touch up every 4 to 8 weeks.

Picking the Right Shade

Just like with clothing, some colors look good on us and some colors don't. When deciding on a hair color, definitely enlist the help of your stylist. If she truly is your BFF, she'll let you know if what you are contemplating is going to make you the belle of the ball or the wicked witch of the west. But just in case, here are a few guidelines:

- Stick to colors that compliment your skin tone. Look at your underlying pigment by turning your hand over and looking at your wrist. Is the skin there pink, peach, olive or yellow?
- Go back to your childhood. Were you blonde as a child? Chances are you'll look great as a blonde adult. If you had light brown hair as a child but your hair as an adult is a mousy, dull, ashy shade, then some caramel or honey highlights might be just the thing.
- Watch out for super dark shades as they can wash you out and make your skin look too harsh or age you.
- Most people can wear red but finding the perfect shade is crucial. Red is where a professional colorist can really earn their keep helping you avoid the wrong choice!
- If you are still undecided, try going to a wig shop and trying on different colors until you find the one that's right for you. Take a

picture in good light so that your stylist can clearly see the color and match it to the hair samples in her color guide.

Care and Maintenance

Now that you have the color that you love, how do you keep it from fading out? First protect your investment with a color protecting shampoo and conditioner. There are lots of professional brands from reputable salons on the market that have UVA and UVB ingredients to protect from the sun and free radicals like dirt and smog that can damage your luscious locks. These products tend to be concentrated and contain higher quality ingredients. Therefore you will be using less and won't have buildup that can cause hair to be limp and flat. When using conditioners be careful to only use them on the ends. Your hair at the root usually doesn't need extra conditioning; it can weigh hair down. Try not to wash your hair everyday, instead just condition and towel dry, but blot don't rub.

Look for a volumizing line for color treated hair. If you have blonde hair or blonde highlights, using a purple shampoo helps tone down any "brassiness." Just don't use it every day or your hair will have a lovely purple hue! A good rule of thumb is to use once a week or whenever you feel that you could use a brightener. Women who have white or silver hair and want to keep it from looking dull or yellow can also use a purple shampoo.

You can sometimes eliminate the damaging effects of pool chemicals by dousing your hair with bottled spring water or using special shampoos designed to minimize the effects of chlorine. And when you have to be in the sun, using a hat in addition to the protective shampoos and conditioners can really keep your color from fading.

Over-processing your hair either chemically or with heat can have catastrophic results. Sometimes the only cure for the worst damage is to cut it off. Fine hair is more susceptible to damage because of the hair shaft being so fragile. It is true that once hair is damaged you can't "un-damage" it, but you can help protect the remaining undamaged hair and prevent it from getting worse. Damaged hair can be repaired over time. Protein treatments work wonders since hair is primarily made out of protein. The treatment aids in rebuilding lost protein. You might also want to help stimulate hair growth by eating a high protein diet and taking supplements like Biotin and fish oil. These are discussed in more detail in Chapter 8. Suffice it to say that proteins help rebuild your hair's amino acids and improve resilience against damage caused by everyday environmental factors and styling.

Try not to use styling tools such as flat irons and curling irons. The intense heat in these devices can strip the hair shaft of moisture. Invest in an ionic blow dryer. It is less damaging, adds shine to your hair and will help it dry a little faster. Also, try not to pull it up into a ponytail. The less you do to your damaged hair the faster you will be on the road to recovery.

THE LITTLE WHITE LIE

So you weren't born with the world's greatest hair. So what? Chances are you weren't born with the world's greatest nose, teeth, nails, or breasts either. But that doesn't hold you back. With today's ever increasing knowledge of science, biology and technology none of us has to live with what nature gave us. From whitening strips to wonder bras, from acrylic nails to a discreet nip/tuck, we can all indulge in the little white lies that make us feel so much better about ourselves. And our hair is no different.

If none of the tips in this book have so far gotten you the fabulous look that you've been yearning for then this chapter is for you! It used to be that wearing "fake" hair was something only done on Halloween or by stage and screen actresses in order to pull off a particular role. Well those days are long gone! Now everyone can, and many, many people do, sport the latest styles without having to change a thing about their natural hair. Celebrities in particular have embraced and glamorized the "extension." From short one day to long and lush the next, celebrities "change" their hairstyles almost as often as they change their underwear. It's become so main stream that we've forgotten the days when only Dolly Parton had the courage to own up to hair that wasn't her own.

Not to mention that hair pieces, i.e. wigs, falls, and extensions are great ways to try a new look, and particularly a new color, without having to make a commitment. Far from looking fake, today's hair pieces look natural and come in numerous shades so you can always find one to match or complement your current hair color. Even the synthetics have been greatly improved to look just like a real head of hair. Application methods and designs have improved as well allowing for greater breathability, comfort and sizing.

<u>Wigs and Falls</u>

Both wigs and falls cover the entire head. The main difference is that a wig adheres to the head with a tight cap while a fall has clamps or combs that attach to the front of the hair line. Falls are also sometimes used to specifically fill in spots where hair is thinning. Because falls use clamps and combs they can be harsh on fine hair. When worn too often traction alopecia may occur. Traction alopecia is a type of hair loss caused by subjecting the hair to excessive pulling force. For this reason, wigs are a better choice for women with fine hair.

Wigs today are made of both human hair and synthetic materials. It used to be that human hair wigs looked more natural but with advancements in materials, synthetic wigs look equally good. The real choice now is convenience.

Synthetic wigs are easy to wear and care for. They generally come pre-styled. Shorter synthetic wigs are called "shake-n-go" meaning all you have to do is shake them out and they look great. Longer wigs require a bit of finger or plastic combing.

The important thing to remember with a synthetic wig is never to use any type of heat around them. Curling irons, flat irons, and even blow dryers on a heat setting will damage the material in the wig.

Human hair wigs on the other hand are just like your own hair and can be treated as such including the use of hot styling tools. They do not come pre-styled and so require the same amount of styling effort that you would use with your own hair. Because they are real hair they tend to weigh a little more.

Contrary to popular belief, wigs will not cause damage to the scalp or slow natural hair growth. In addition to boosting the confidence and self-esteem of some women, wigs can also be used to help maintain body heat and to prevent over-exposure of sensitive skin to the elements. Hate wearing a ball cap in the summer to prevent your scalp from burning? Try a lightweight wig instead! Wish you could ride around all day in a convertible and still have your fine hair look fabulous and not tangled? A wig might be the answer. Match one to your natural color and style and you'll be good to go!

Make sure you care for your wig as you would your own hair. Only use professional hair care products designed specifically for wigs. The same goes for your styling tools. Avoid using a standard hair brush as they can overstretch and damage the wig. Always start from the hair end when brushing a wig and work up to the root. At the end of the day, place your wig on a Styrofoam stand. Refrain from sleeping in your wig unless absolutely necessary. The tossing and turning you do as you sleep could pull on the wig where the hair is attached to the cap and cause damage effectively reducing the life of the wig.

Extensions

If you want to achieve a temporary change in your look then extensions may be the way to go. Extensions have become very popular as witnessed by the many celebrities who have created their own brands. But extensions are not for everyone and those of us with fine or thin hair should be extremely careful. The methods for adhering extensions can do more harm than good with our hair types. In some cases bald spots can result that do not grow back because the extension pulled on the root of the hair and damaged the follicle. It is critical that you find a stylist who is very experienced in working with extensions and fine hair before you go down this path. That person may not be the same stylist who does your hair normally. Don't allow yourself to become one of the many horror stories of extensions done badly.

As with wigs, extensions may be made from human hair or synthetics. But unlike wigs that simply fit over your head, extensions have to be attached in one way or another to your natural hair. In some attachment methods a glue or bond is used that involves coating your hair with a chemical. Ask your stylist in advance if any chemicals will be used and try to determine if you may have a harmful reaction to them.

In general there are 3 types of extension processes:

1. <u>Strand by strand</u>: in this process small strands of hair are attached one by one to small sections of your own hair by either weaving in, gluing, heat fusing, clamping with metal tubes or using waxes and polymers.

2. <u>Weft</u>: an extension composed of a track of several inches long on which hair is already attached. Think of it as the cross fibers in a piece of cloth. The hair is tight together at the top and free flowing at the bottom. The track extension is then sewn to a corn row braid of your natural hair that extends from ear to ear along the back of your head.

3. <u>Clip-in</u>: as the name implies these hair extensions are attached to clips. You simply clip them in where you want and remove them at the end of the day before bed. Clip-ins are the fun way to go from short to long and back again with the least amount of fuss.

Hair extensions will last between 2 and 6 months depending on the method used and the brand of extension. This is due mainly to the growth of your own hair but sometimes may be because the attachment breaks. As extensions get loose they need to be removed or retightened. This should only be done by a professional as solvents are needed. You may be able to reuse some of the hair and keep your cost down if you start with a high quality product and take good care of it. Consult your stylist on exactly how to wash your hair, dry it and style it. It is important to avoid tangling and matting as much as possible to extend the life of your extensions.

YOU'RE NOT LOSING YOUR HAIR – IT'S RIGHT IN YOUR BRUSH!

So, you woke up, looked in the mirror and held your breath, sure you had lost another hair. Had you taken the wrong medicine, too much stress, vitamin deficiency, hormones? What was the culprit this time? You swear to yourself you're going to start counting your hairs every morning. **Breathe**.

While it is true that many of these things can cause hair loss, there are things you can do to treat, prevent, or hide hair loss. No need to panic before weighing your options.

Diet and Nutrition

Vitamins and diet can play a vital part in hair restoration. And the best part is that it they won't cost you an arm and a leg. It has been shown that certain vitamin deficiencies can cause hair to become fine and thin or fall out. So before pulling out your magnifying glass to start counting, try supplementing a few vitamins known to assist in hair growth. Malnourishment is also known to cause hair loss, so eating plenty of healthy foods is a key to healthy hair. Have you heard the saying, you can see your health through your hair? Well it's true. If your body feels all shiny and bouncy then you stand a much better chance that your hair will too.

As in all things moderation is often the key to success. So don't read this chapter and then go buy out the first health store you come to. Finding the right supplements for your needs is necessary before beginning any regimen. Your body will try to flush out toxins whatever way it can. Too many vitamins and minerals could lead to opposite than intended effects.

As always with any supplement or vitamin you should consult your physician, start out small and add as recommended. Particularly if you are taking other medications as some could have adverse reactions when taken together.

One of the more popular natural treatments to save your hair is biotin. Biotin, part of the B vitamins cluster, is so strongly recommended that it is usually one of the first supplements suggested to hair loss patients. Biotin can be found in several foods, but not in the large doses needed by the body. Taking a supplement to increase your biotin intake is one giant leap towards healthier hair. Biotin is sold in dosages of 2500 to 5000 mg. It is suggested to take 2500 mg and attempt to supplement the rest through foods such as liver (or other organ meats), cauliflower, salmon, bananas, carrots and egg yolks. Sardines are also high in biotin, and they have been rumored to "put hair on your chest" so I guess the head can't be far behind. **Biotin supplement is not considered safe for seizure patients.**

Another common remedy is increasing iron intake. Iron is known to be beneficial in many ways. Approximately ten percent of your iron intake is actually absorbed into your body and blood stream. To put it in perspective that's like getting a chocolate chip cookie and only being able to eat the chips! The rest goes to waste. Of course there are foods that are rich in iron to help give you a small boost such as, red meat (vegetarians, don't panic), leafy greens (see, all better), shellfish, eggs (known as the super food for hair), oranges (or any other vitamin C filled foods), and nuts and grains. When our body starts losing iron, it loses essential energy to properly perform its functions. Then it begins to pick and choose which bodily functions are more important and begins minimizing energy consuming tasks. As much as we ladies may want to disagree, our bodies just cannot be convinced that growing our hair really *is* more important than our bone marrow!

There are also foods that exasperate iron deficiencies. You know how most diets tell you to only eat the egg white and throw out the yolk? Unfortunately, it is the egg yolk that provides most of the nutrition and protein needed for hair health. The egg white offers a different type of protein called albumin that can decrease the body's ability to absorb needed iron. Bran, coffee and tea are also strong enemies to the absorption of iron. Coffee lovers don't scream! The trick is drinking water, milk, or juice with meals and saving soft drinks, coffee and tea for a later time after meals have been digested.

A healthy diet filled with fresh foods is a key to guaranteeing proper nutrition. While counting ice cream as your daily dairy serving may taste better, the lack of vitamins and minerals makes it an empty snack with no hair benefits. But eating foods rich in vitamins E, D, A and C encourage hair growth from the root to the tip. Adding adequate servings of protein into your diet has been said to increase energy, improve mood, and reduce hair loss. Protein is also believed to be necessary for the body to repair effectively. Foods that offer ample protein are liver, egg yolks (remember super hair food right?), nuts, chicken and soy.

Consuming a variety of fruits and vegetables provides essential vitamins and minerals such as Folic acid, vitamin C, Vitamin B6 and B12 just to name a few. They provide your body with the proper nutrition to enhance hair growth through stimulating the scalp, encouraging cell growth, and strengthening the hair follicles. Vitamin C is not only an excellent antioxidant, but also increases the blood flow to the scalp. Dark leafy greens are rich in vitamin C and vitamin E, which is known to add strength and shine to your hair. They also contain the antioxidant that increases scalp stimulation. Cruciferous vegetables, peppers, and squash are high in vitamins C and E, are low in fat, and low in carbohydrates making them the perfect foods to incorporate into your meals.

There are conflicting studies of the effects of using a low carbohydrate diet plan. There is some evidence that for those whose hair loss is related to issues surrounding hypoglycemia, a low carbohydrate diet can be beneficial. For those with no glucose problems, however, low carbohydrate diets have been shown to be responsible for causing the opposite effect. Once again, too much of a good thing, is never a good thing. The believed cause of hair loss in this instance is the high protein counter to the low carbohydrate diet. While the body may need protein to function, your kidneys can't process more than the recommended serving before causing complications. It is also common belief that hair loss occurs when on low carbohydrate diets due to the strict food restrictions. If all you are feeding your body is protein, it isn't getting any of the other nutrients it needs. This leads to -

you guessed it - vitamin and mineral deficiencies.

Hair Growth Products

While foods and vitamins and natural remedies are a great start to maintaining hair thickness or minimizing loss there are other options available. Rogaine® is a popular treatment for women suffering hair loss. Its main ingredient, Minoxidil, is also the **only** medication approved by the Federal Drug Administration. Minoxidil was originally created and tested for patients with hypertensive issues.

While it successfully lowered blood pressure, it also caused increased hair growth in its users. When tested in liquid form on the scalp it was shown to hold the same effect. This can help boost a woman's self esteem, give her back her confidence, while improving mood stability. **Please note that while the key ingredient was once used in oral medication, this product is in no way safe for internal use.**

Rogaine® can be beneficial to your regimen if you are suffering specific types of hair loss. Women with hereditary hair loss benefit most from the use of Rogaine®. Those with patchy hair loss, no familial history of hair loss, or sudden hair loss possibly accompanied by an irritated red scalp should not use this product. There are also dangers with taking this medication if you suffer from any type of cardiac disease so **be sure to check with your doctor before using.** One of the largest downfalls of medications like Rogaine® is the abruptness in which you stop growing hair and start losing it again if you are forced to stop treatment. This is true even if the interruption to treatment is minimal. Rogaine®, in this way, becomes a life sentence of paying out large sums of money for hair restoration. If you are willing to take the risk of possible side effects and use the product faithfully, it is a definite proven remedy for hair loss.

Spironolactone is a water pill that also acts as a treatment for women with thinning hair. It works by slowing down the production of androgens in the glands and ovaries. Cimetidine, another popular medication specified for women is commonly used for treatment of symptoms related to polycystic ovary syndrome or PCOS. Cimetidine, originally used as a histamine blocker to alleviate ulcers, has now shown to harbor a strong anti-androgenic property. Also aiding in the hair restoration process is its power to block dehydrotestosterone, one of the causes of hair loss, from banding with its androgenic partner.

Hair Growth Treatments

Low light laser therapy is quickly becoming a popular treatment option to women with thinning hair. This option, now available at home with the purchase of a laser comb, uses low light being spread across the scalp in an effort to inundate the cells with energy promoting hair growth. Traditionally offered in salons for several treatments a month over the course of a year, the technique has been recently modified to a more user friendly version.

While proving an increase in hair growth and strength, this method is often argued against in favor of hair transplants. The reason for this is the lack of substantial hair growth while using the laser comb versus almost total restoration using the transplant method. While laser combs also benefit all around hair health, it is evident that actual hair re-growth is minimal when using this product.

Hair transplants are one of the most common treatments for hair loss in women. This treatment is becoming more popular due to the effectiveness and length of time it lasts. Hair transplant consists of taking healthy follicles from the back of the scalp, and placing it where hair thinning or baldness is the greatest. When done correctly, this method allows natural looking hair that will re-grow several times with minimal scarring. If the transplant takes, the hair that is restored will last for a long period of time before the follicles fail.

While proving excellent results when hair transplant takes, it is not without cost or risk. When looking at average total costs for hair restoration, transplants are generally less than or equal to other treatments in the long run. The reason it seems so much more expensive is because it is generally paid in one lump sum or several large payments at once. The good news is several facilities now offer payment plans to assist with the costs of surgery. And the results can be lifelong eliminating the need to spend money on other treatments.

Hair transplants often have to be repeated several times for optimal effect and desired thickness. This not only adds to the cost, but also adds to the time involved in the treatment as six months is required between each transplant. If you choose this method be cautious of setting your expectations too high and setting yourself up for disappointment. Transplants can only improve the amount of hair. They will not give your hair a different texture since you are "transplanting" your own hair follicles from one part of your head to another. Thus you will not emerge from the operation with that TV model look we talked about in Chapter 2.

When deciding whether or not hair transplant is the right choice for you consider the health risks involved as well. Surgery, no matter what type always carries some danger. Swelling, tenderness, infections, and unexpected problems can come up during any surgery, including hair restoration surgeries.

When realizing you are beginning to lose hair, it can be difficult not to immediately hit panic mode. The truth is there are many studies working on even better ways to improve hair restoration. Some promising methods are getting really close to making it out on the market. Our hair is a source of pride for us and it can be tough to watch it go down the drain. There are few things that will strike fear or panic in a woman faster than looking in the mirror and seeing those traces of pink scalp.

Just remember there are several options available and talking to your doctor to pinpoint your specific type of hair loss can start you on the right road to recovery. Stress can increase hair loss as well, so get out the bubble bath, turn on your favorite tunes and relax knowing you are working hard at keeping and growing hair.

ABOUT THE AUTHORS

Caren Cantrell is a former bank executive turned author and publisher. She became a client of Melissa's after moving to Scottsdale from Ohio where she had used the same stylist for over 20 years. Caren also has thin, fine hair and had tried several other stylists before finding Melissa and the secrets to looking fabulous. Determined to help other women with similar issues, this book was born while in Melissa's chair between cuts and colors.

Melissa Glass is a hair care extraordinaire who specializes in working with fine, thin hair. Born with fine hair herself, she has dedicated her professional career to helping women solve their styling problems regardless of hair type.